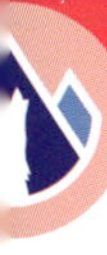

MAJOR DISASTERS

COVID-19

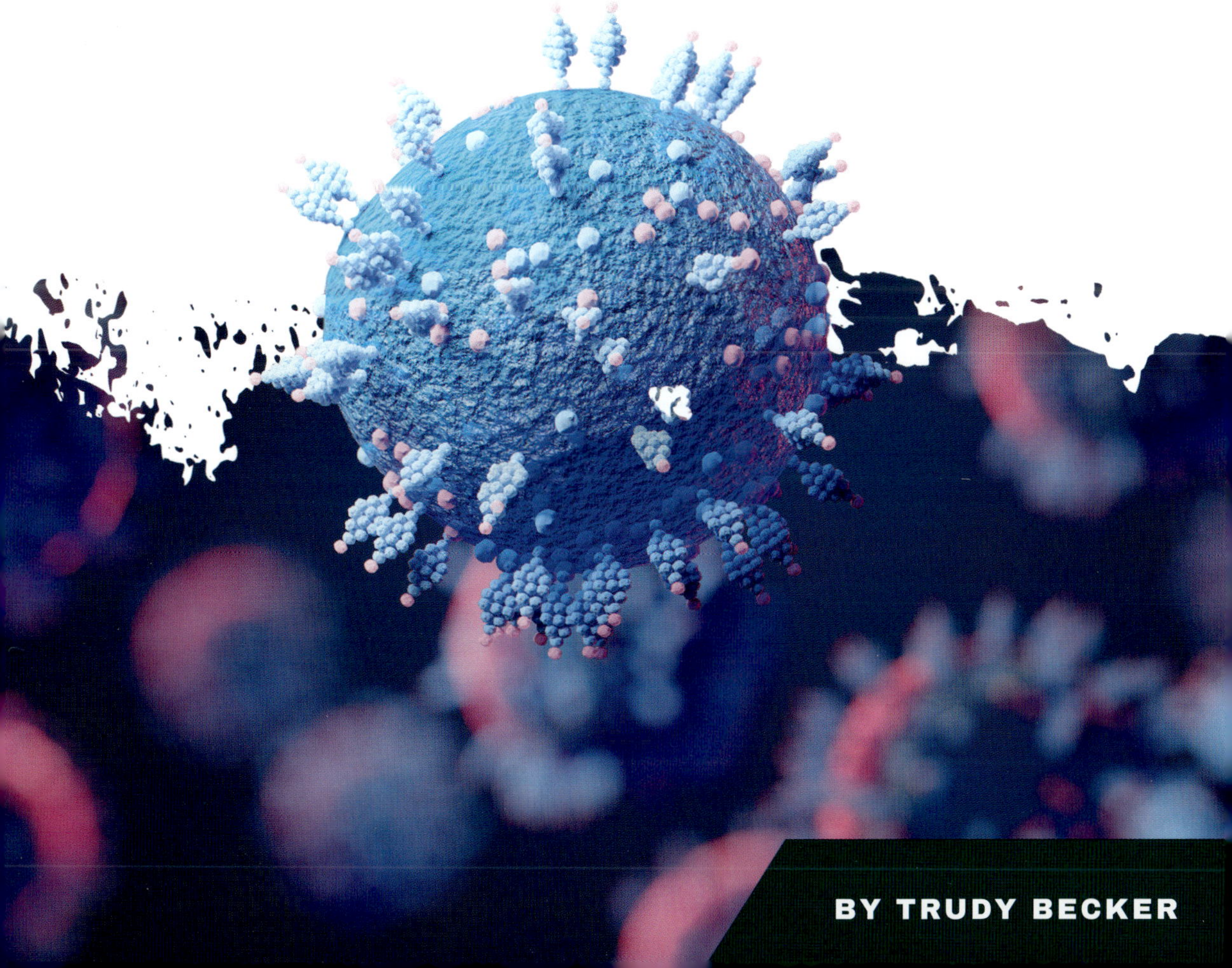

BY TRUDY BECKER

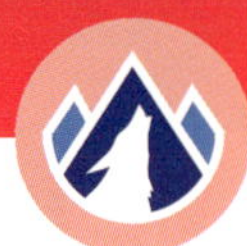

WWW.APEXEDITIONS.COM

Apex is distributed by North Star Editions:
sales@northstareditions.com | 888-417-0195

Produced for Apex by Red Line Editorial.

Photographs ©: Shutterstock Images, cover, 1, 4–5, 6, 7, 12, 15, 16–17, 19, 22–23, 24, 25, 26–27, 29; iStockphoto, 8–9, 13; Yuan Zheng/FeatureChina/AP Images, 10–11; Deividi Correa/Estadao Conteudo/Agencia Estado/AP Images, 14; Jim Mone/AP Images, 18; Kevin C. Cox/Getty Images/AP Images, 20–21

Library of Congress Control Number: 2023910173

ISBN
978-1-63738-755-9 (hardcover)
978-1-63738-798-6 (paperback)
978-1-63738-881-5 (ebook pdf)
978-1-63738-841-9 (hosted ebook)

Printed in the United States of America
Mankato, MN
012024

NOTE TO PARENTS AND EDUCATORS

Apex books are designed to build literacy skills in striving readers. Exciting, high-interest content attracts and holds readers' attention. The text is carefully leveled to allow students to achieve success quickly. Additional features, such as bolded glossary words for difficult terms, help build comprehension.

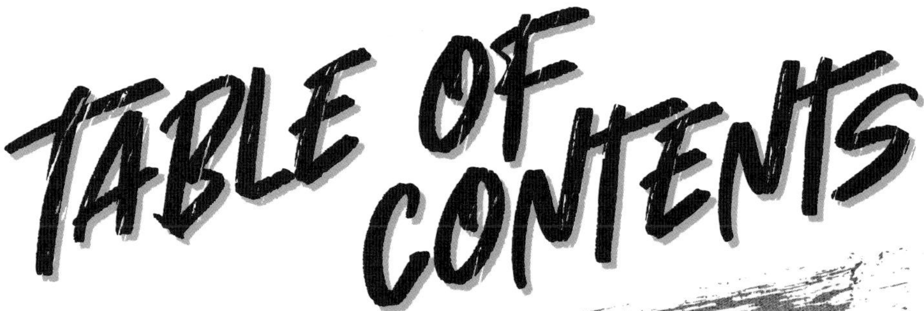
TABLE OF CONTENTS

CHAPTER 1

FEELING SICK

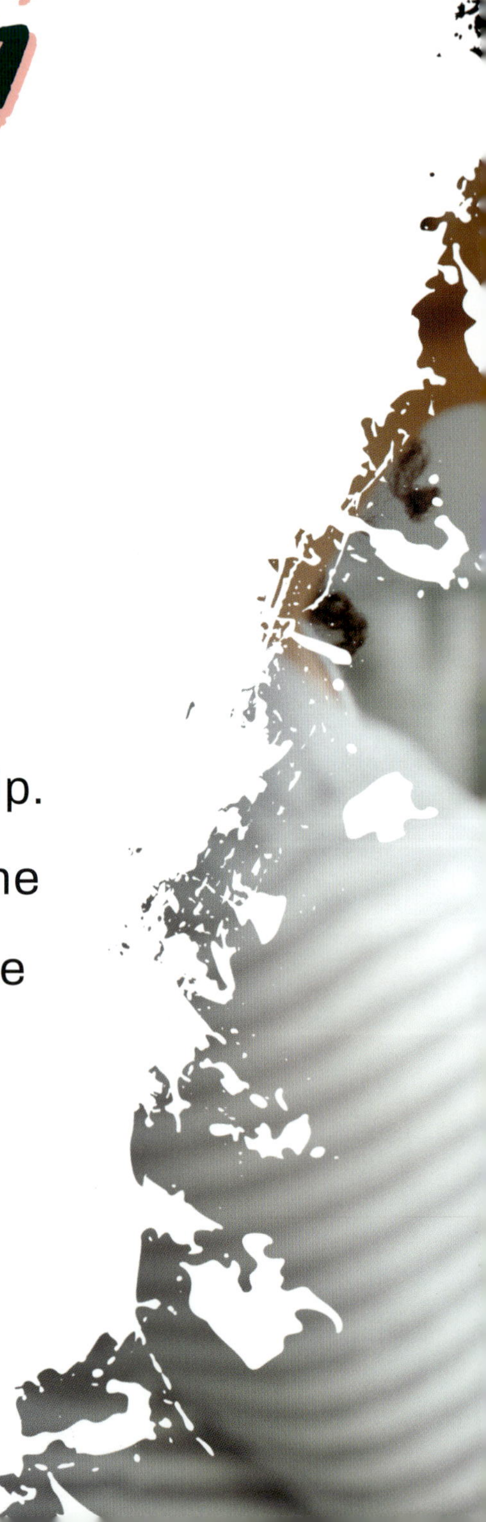

It's mid-2020. A girl arrives home from a trip. She doesn't feel good. She has chills and a fever. She also loses her senses of taste and smell.

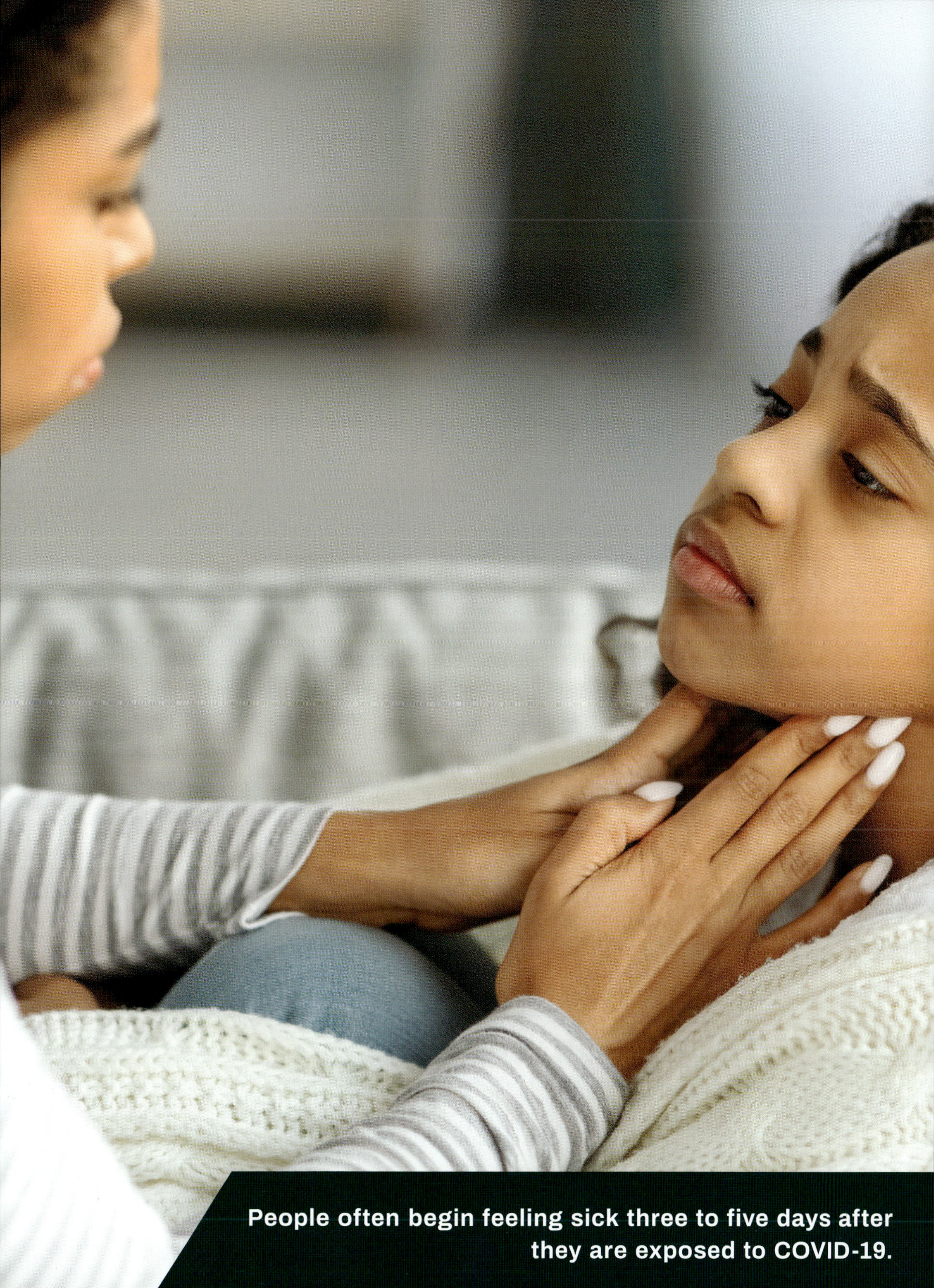

People often begin feeling sick three to five days after they are exposed to COVID-19.

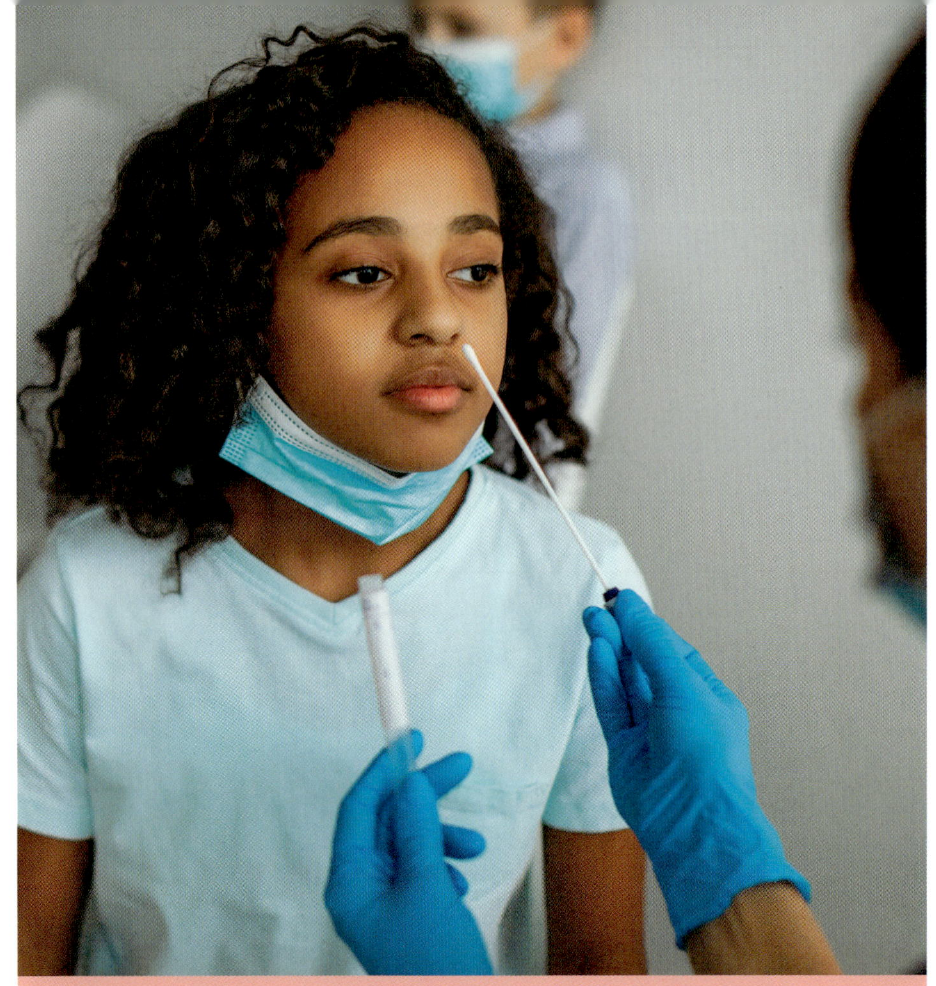

Some tests for COVID-19 use a nose swab. Others use a person's spit.

The girl recognizes these **symptoms**. They may be from COVID-19. So, she goes to a clinic for a test.

FAST FACT
Some COVID-19 tests give results in just a few minutes.

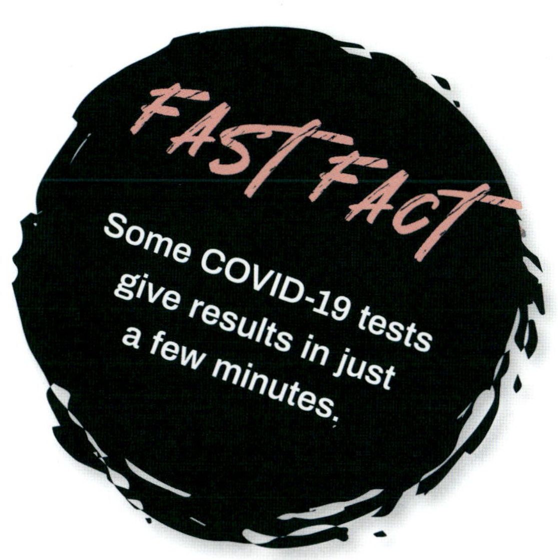

Tests tell people if their symptoms are caused by COVID-19 or by another illness.

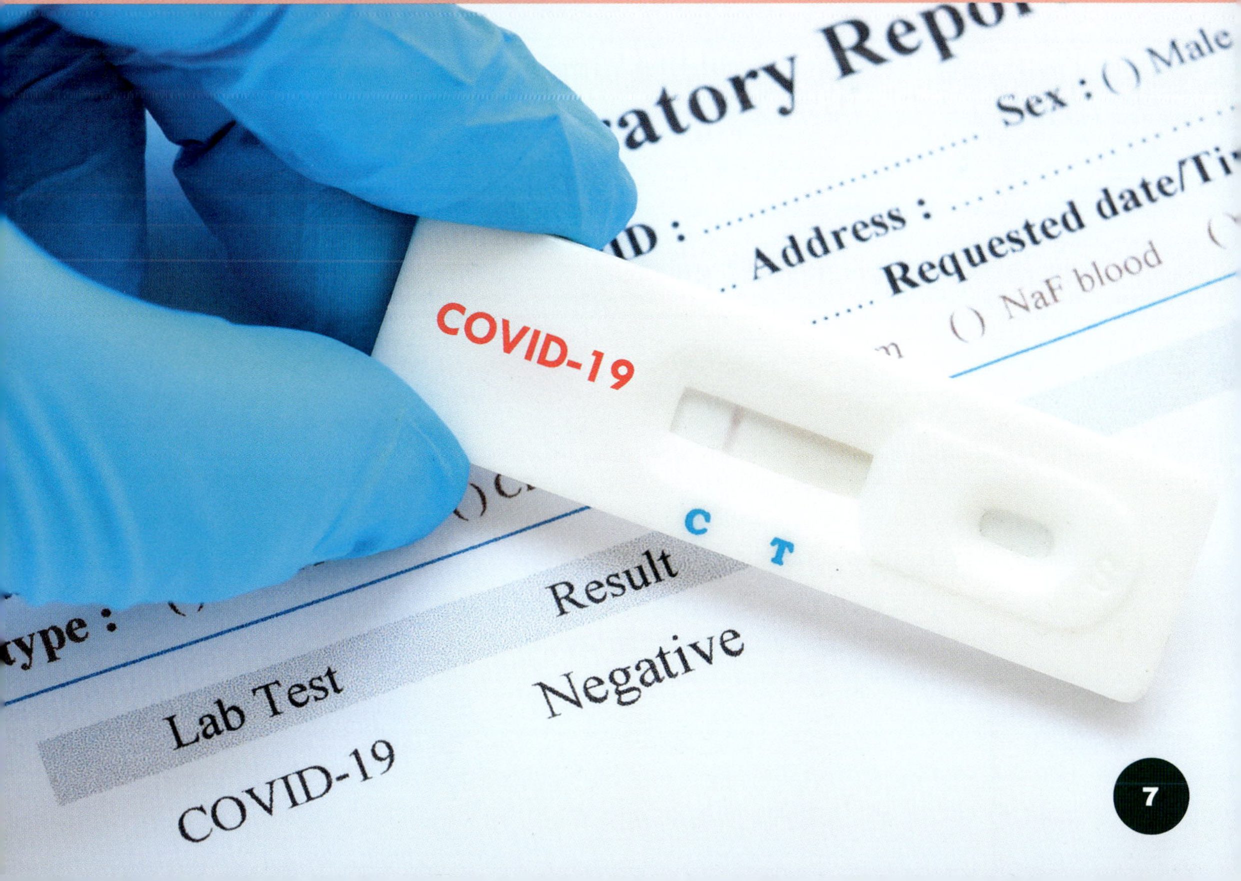

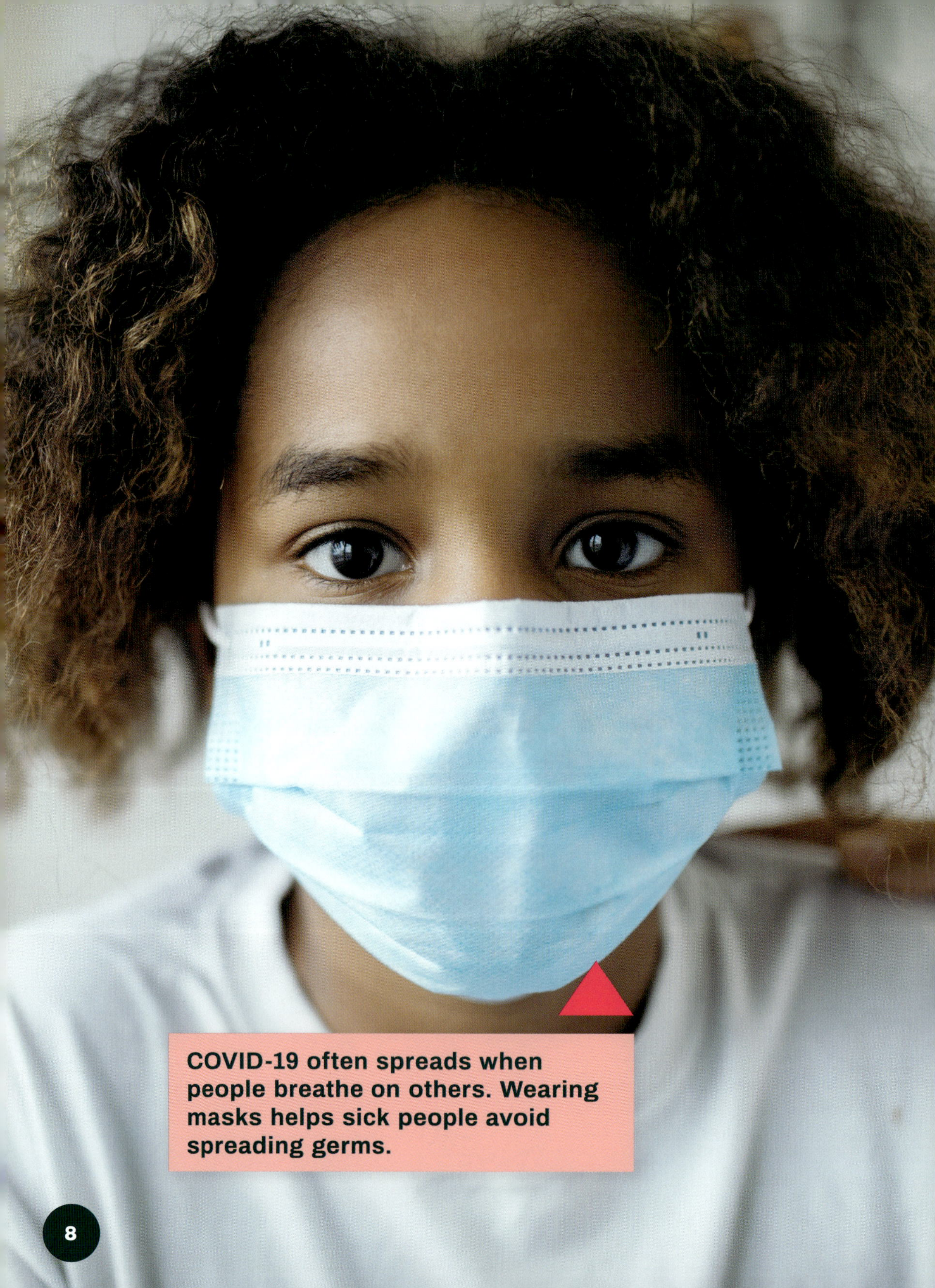

COVID-19 often spreads when people breathe on others. Wearing masks helps sick people avoid spreading germs.

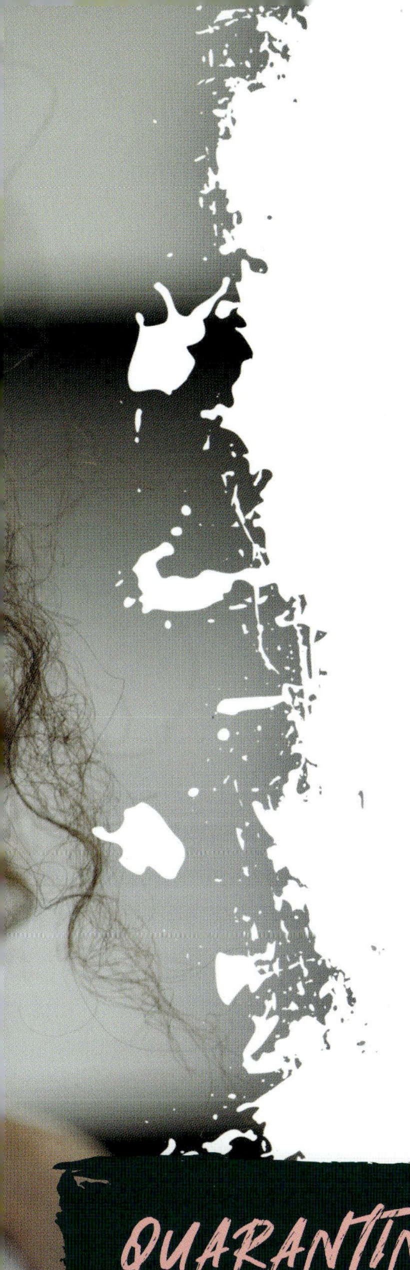

The test is positive. That means the girl has COVID-19. So, she stays home and rests. She wears a mask and stays away from others.

QUARANTINE

Infectious diseases can spread quickly. To slow the spread, people can quarantine. They stay away from other people. That way, fewer people get **exposed**.

CHAPTER 2

GLOBAL DISASTER

COVID-19 is caused by a **virus**. People first noticed it around Wuhan, China, in 2019. The virus quickly spread across the world.

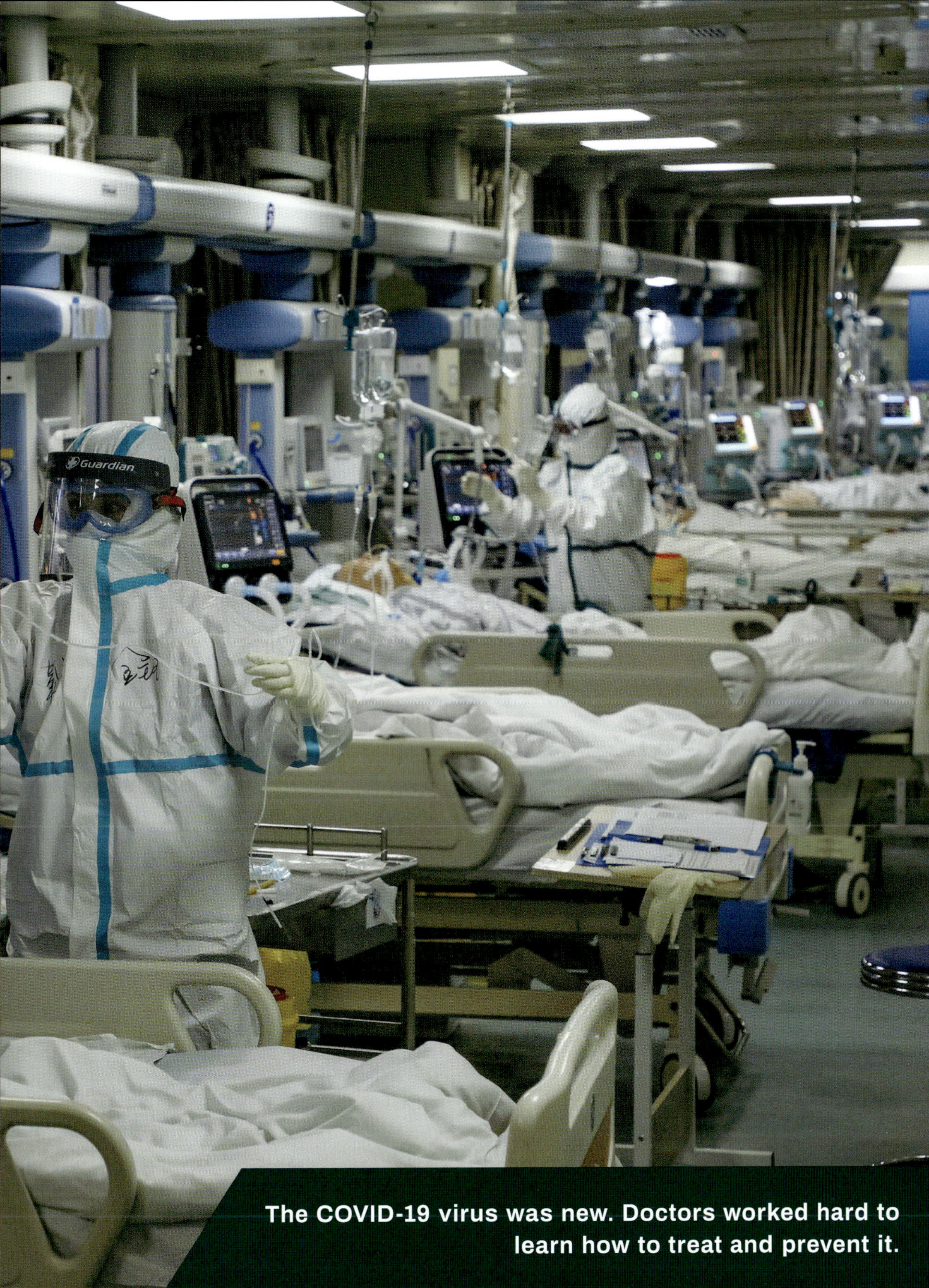

The COVID-19 virus was new. Doctors worked hard to learn how to treat and prevent it.

Many people became sick. By March 2020, COVID-19 was a **pandemic**. Governments limited travel. Schools went online. Many in-person events were canceled.

During 2020, some stores and restaurants had to close. Others had limited hours.

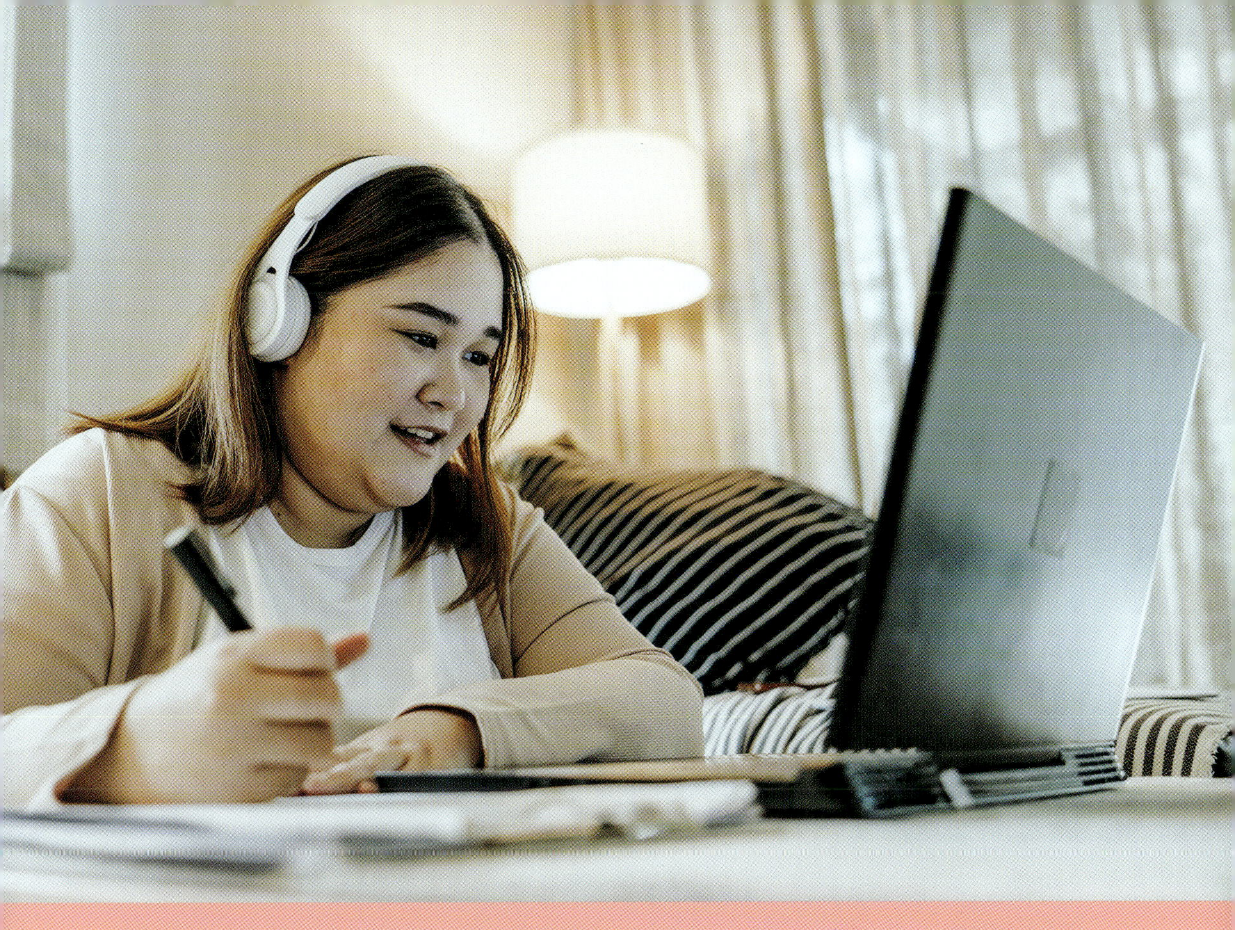

To avoid spreading COVID-19, people stayed home. Many events and classes took place online.

ESSENTIAL WORKERS

Many cities and countries had **lockdowns**. But places like grocery stores and hospitals had to stay open. **Essential** workers helped keep them running. They went to work even during lockdowns.

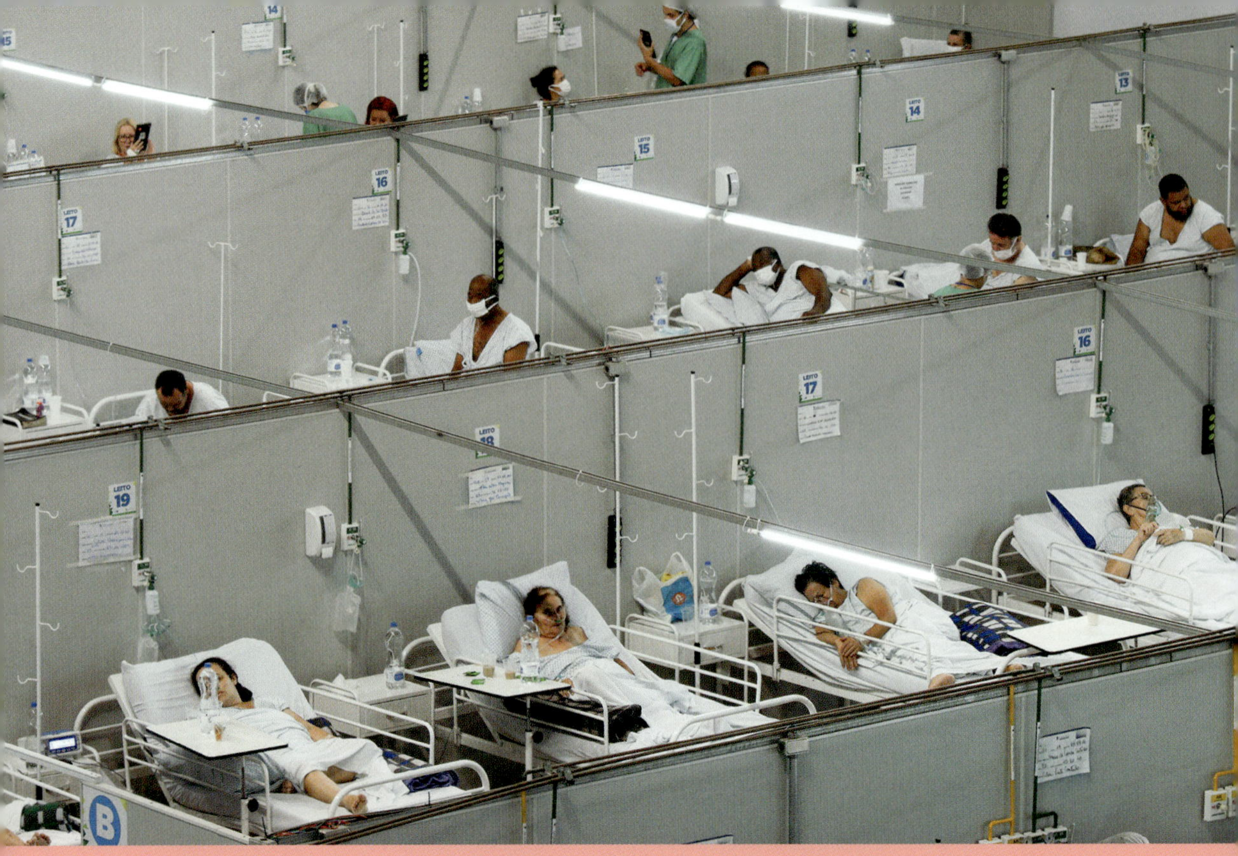

Some cities had to build new hospitals to hold all their patients.

Many people practiced social distancing. They stayed at least 6 feet (2 m) apart. They also wore masks and washed their hands often. Still, the number of cases stayed high for years.

FAST FACT

During 2020, some hospitals became too full. They ran out of space and supplies.

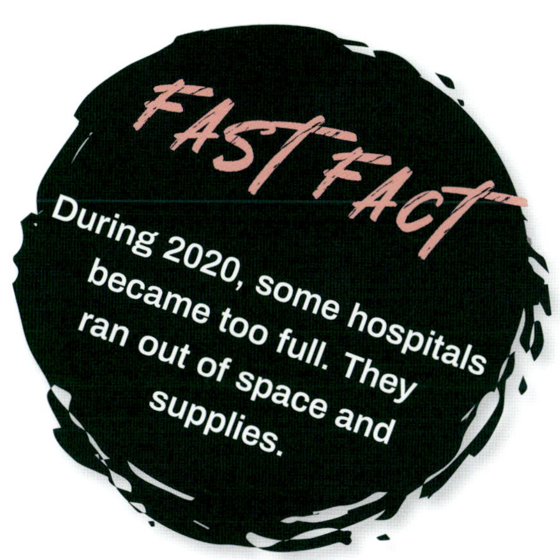

Older people were more likely to get dangerously sick or die.

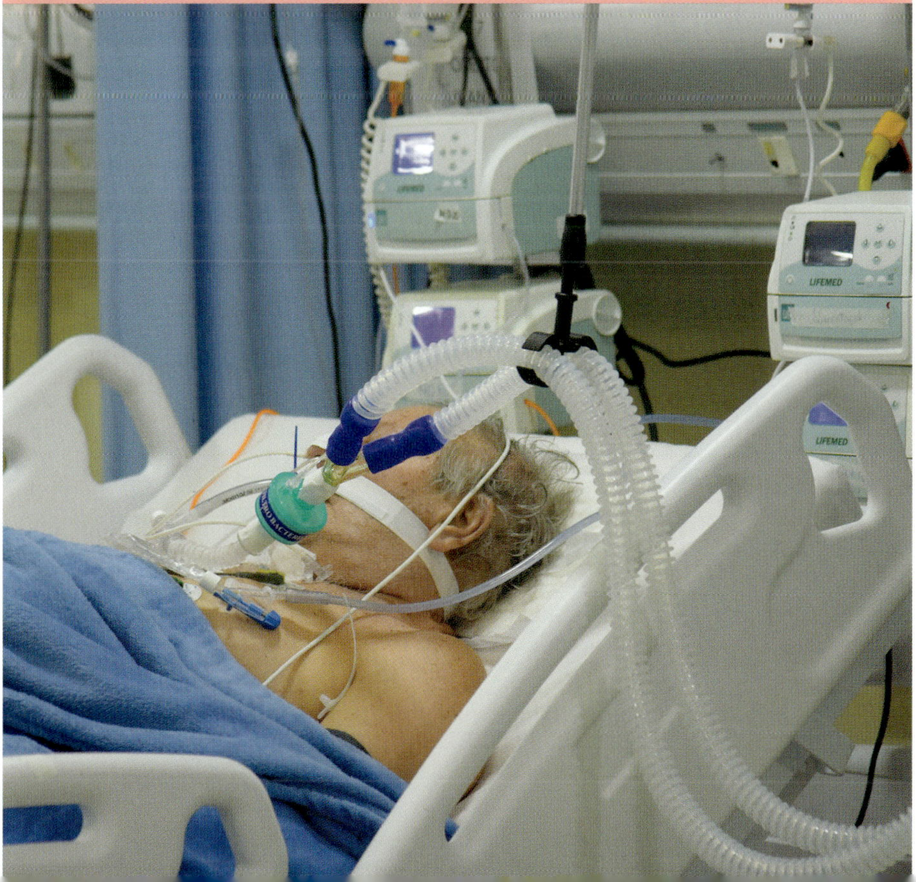

CHAPTER 3

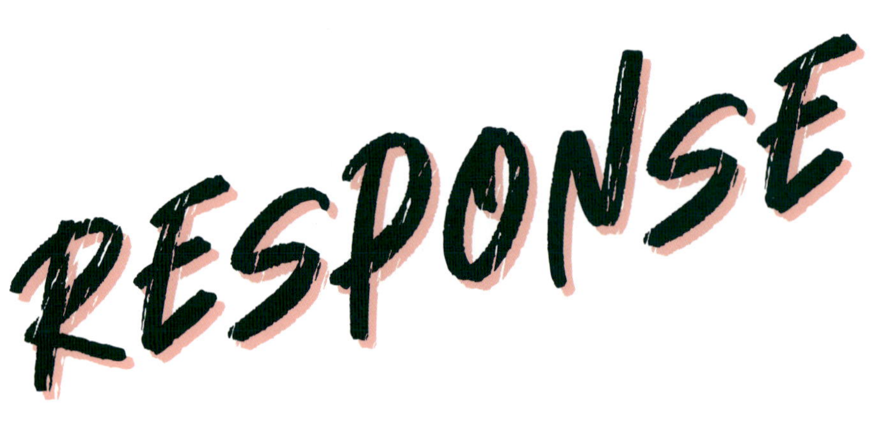

Testing and tracking helped scientists study COVID-19. They used the data to learn more about the virus. This helped them make plans to slow its spread.

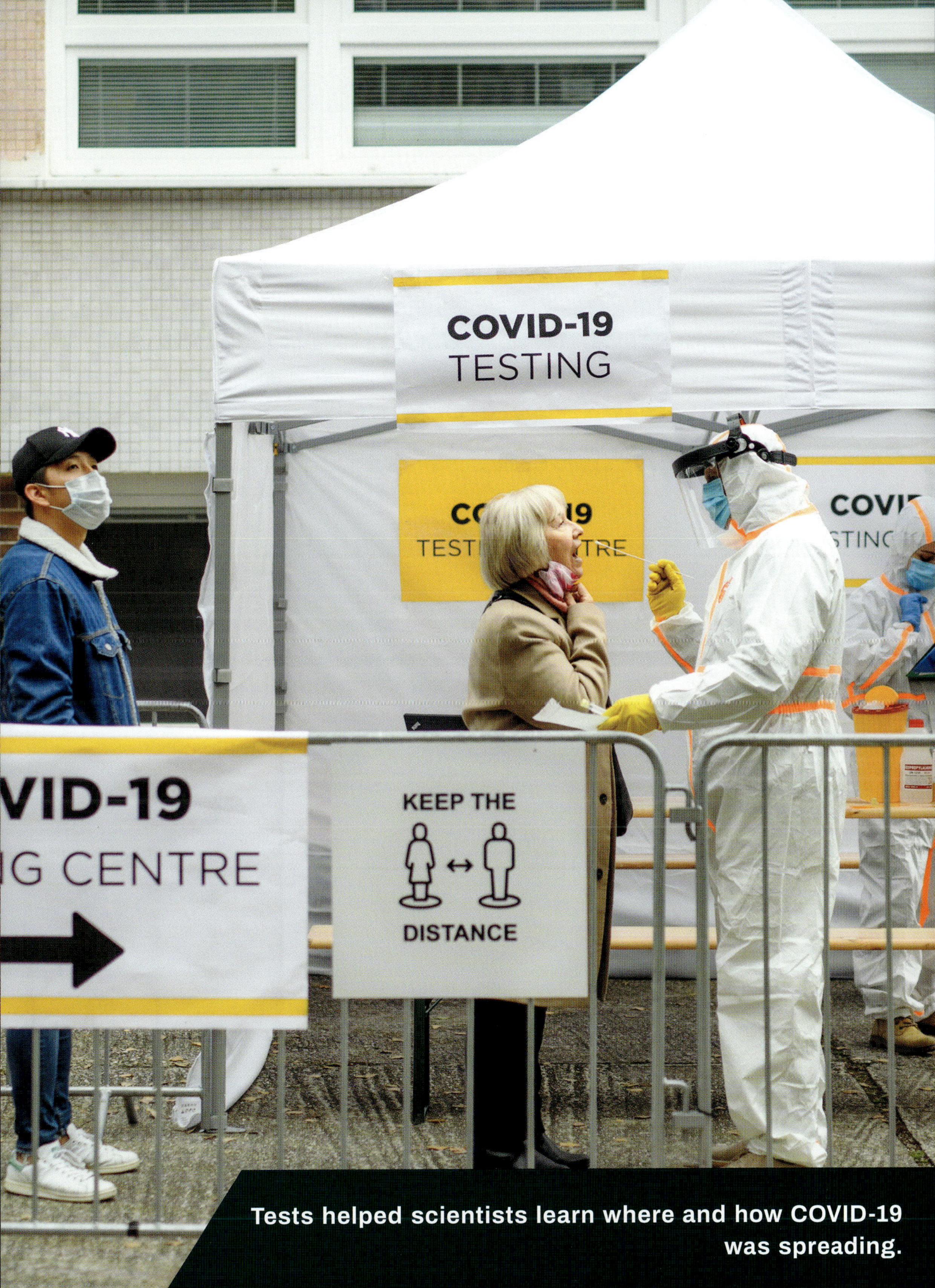

Tests helped scientists learn where and how COVID-19 was spreading.

Vaccines helped, too. Scientists used old and new research to create COVID-19 vaccines. By December 2020, the first vaccines were ready. People got them as shots.

Vaccinated people could still get COVID-19. But they were much less likely to have bad symptoms.

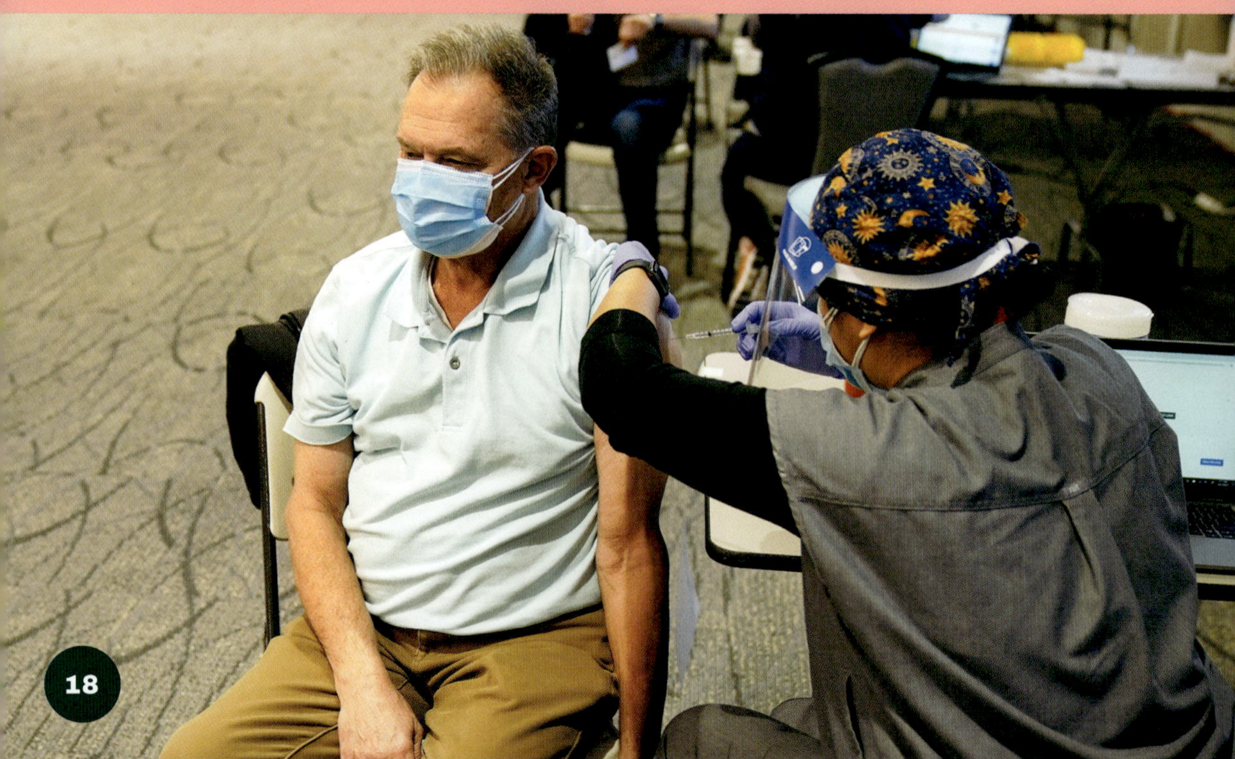

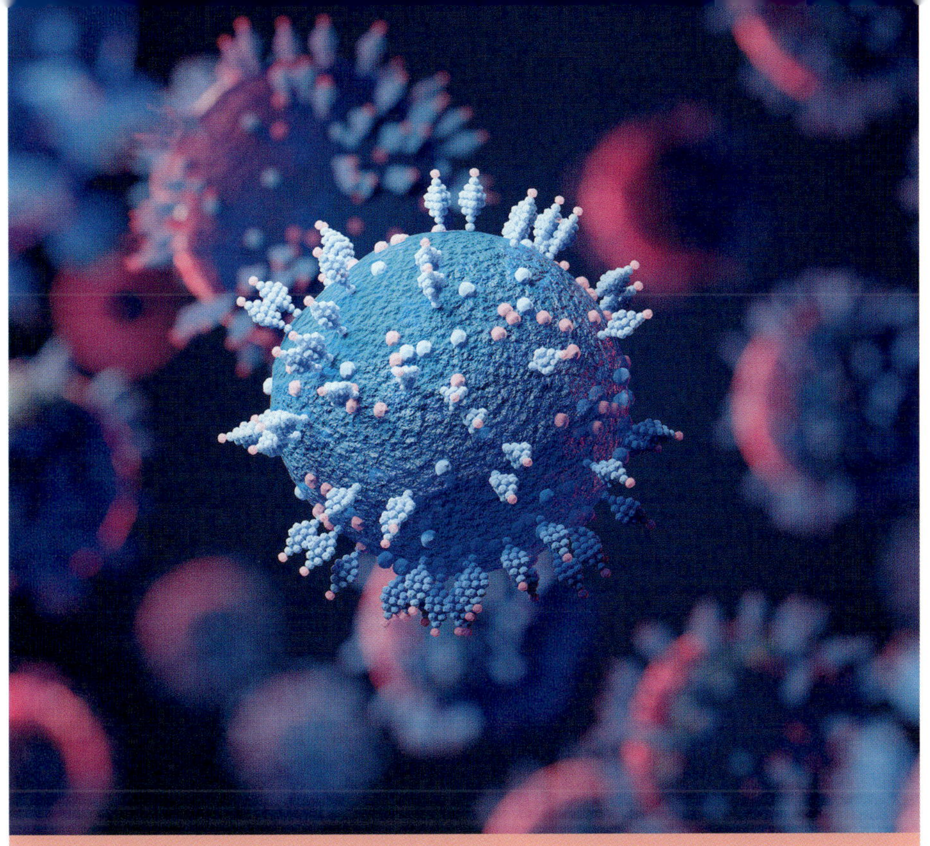

Variants happen when part of a virus changes shape.

NEW VERSIONS

Every virus has a certain shape. Sometimes, this shape changes. The new versions are called variants. COVID-19 had several variants. Some spread faster. They also made people more or less sick.

Gradually, places opened back up. Schools reopened. Events and sports leagues restarted. Numbers of new COVID-19 deaths went down.

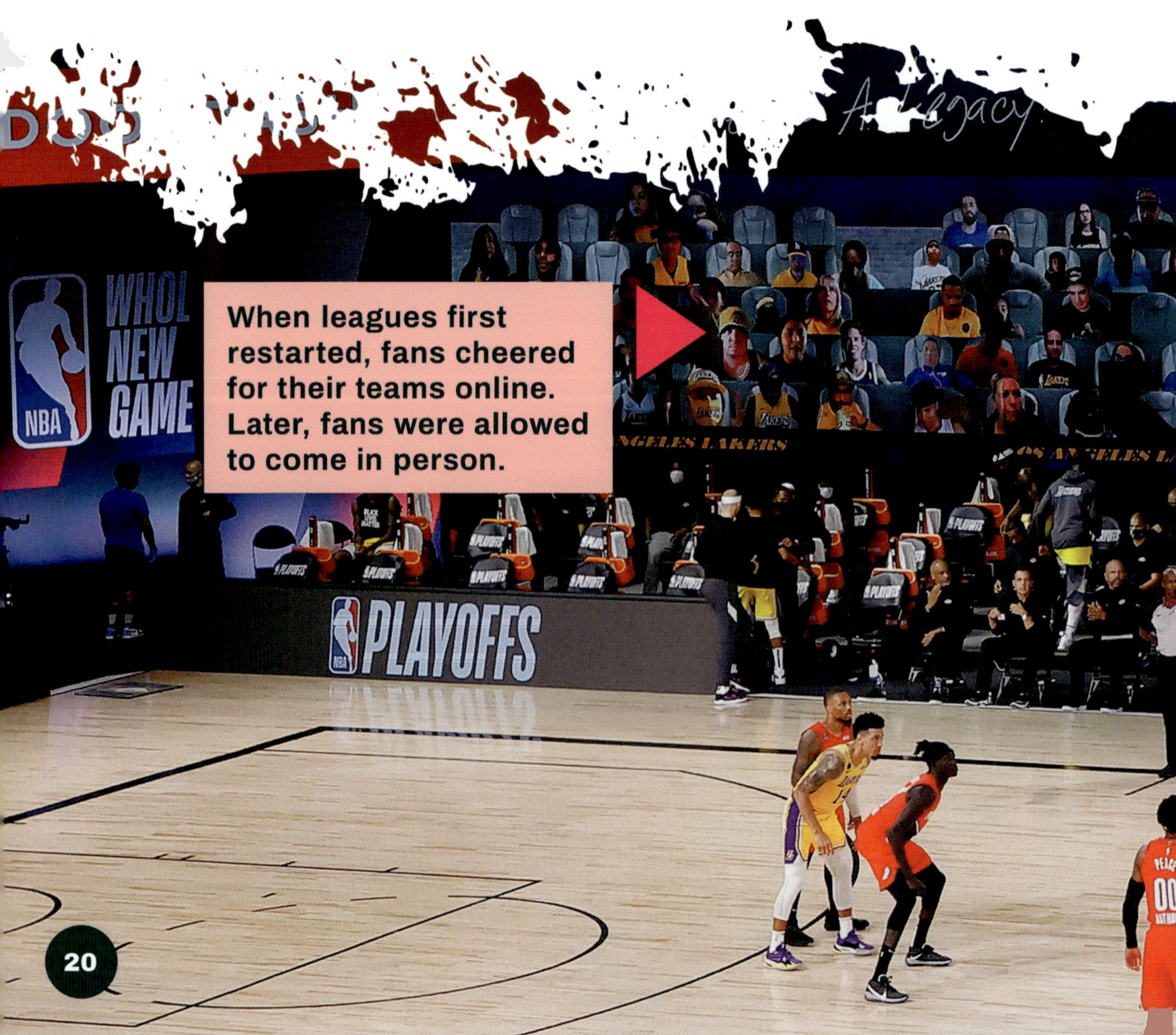

When leagues first restarted, fans cheered for their teams online. Later, fans were allowed to come in person.

FAST FACT

COVID-19 was the worst pandemic in more than 100 years.

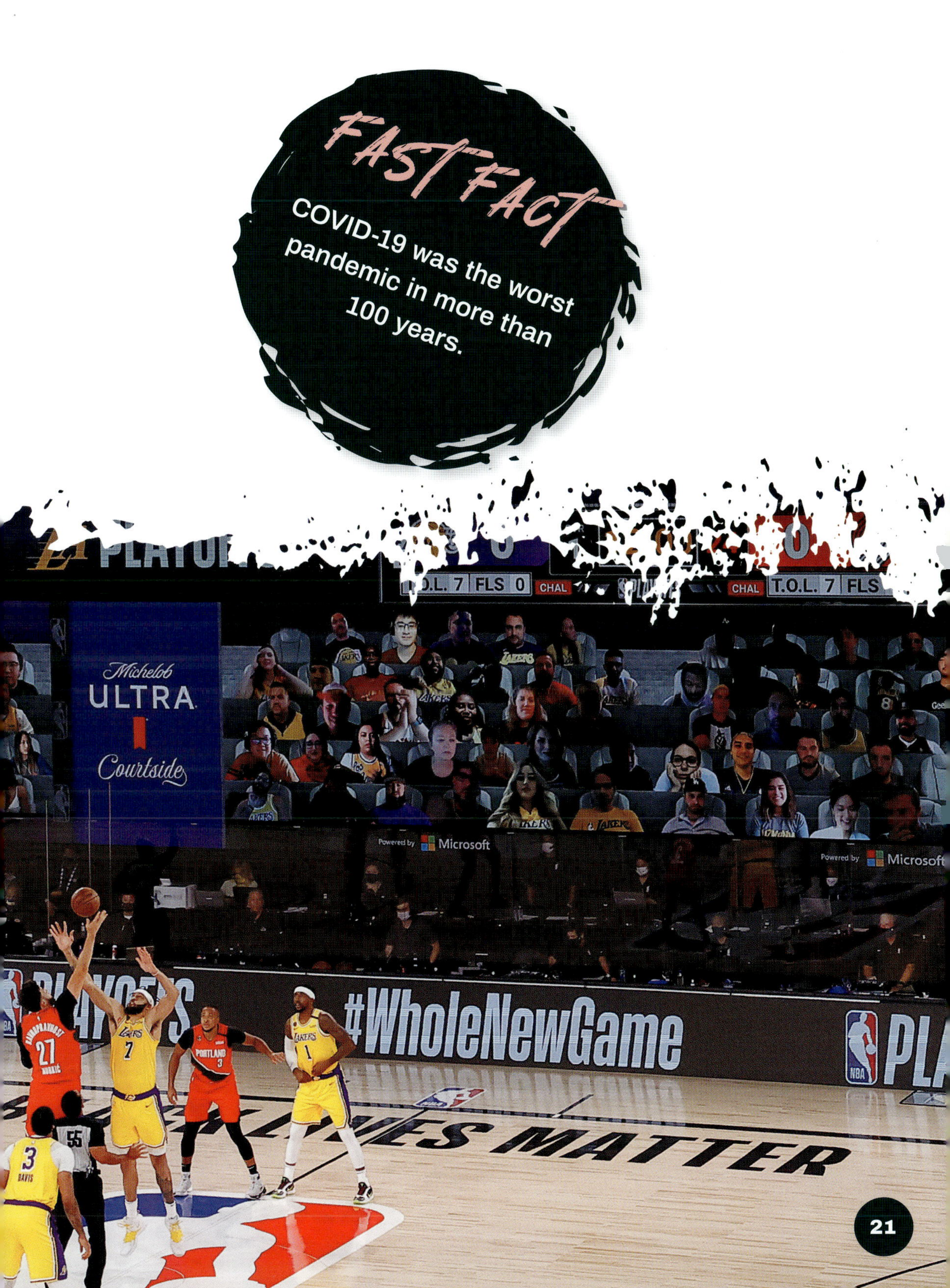

CHAPTER 4

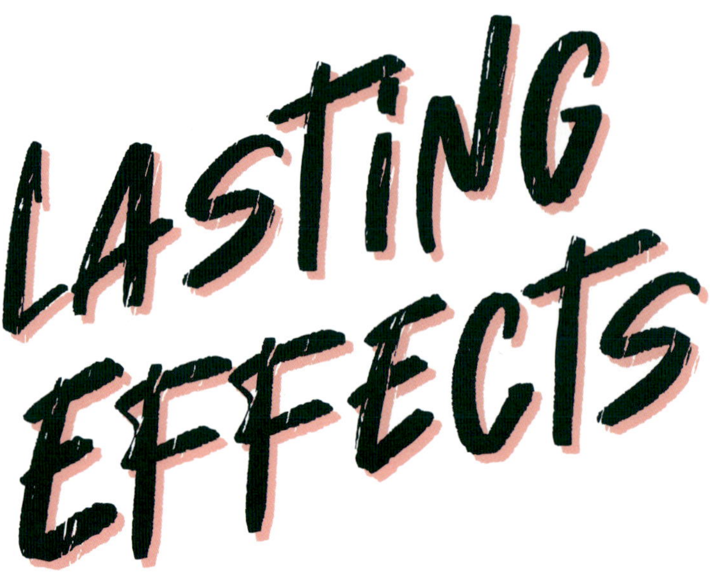

LASTING EFFECTS

COVID-19 had many lasting impacts. During lockdowns, many companies lost money. Millions of people lost their jobs.

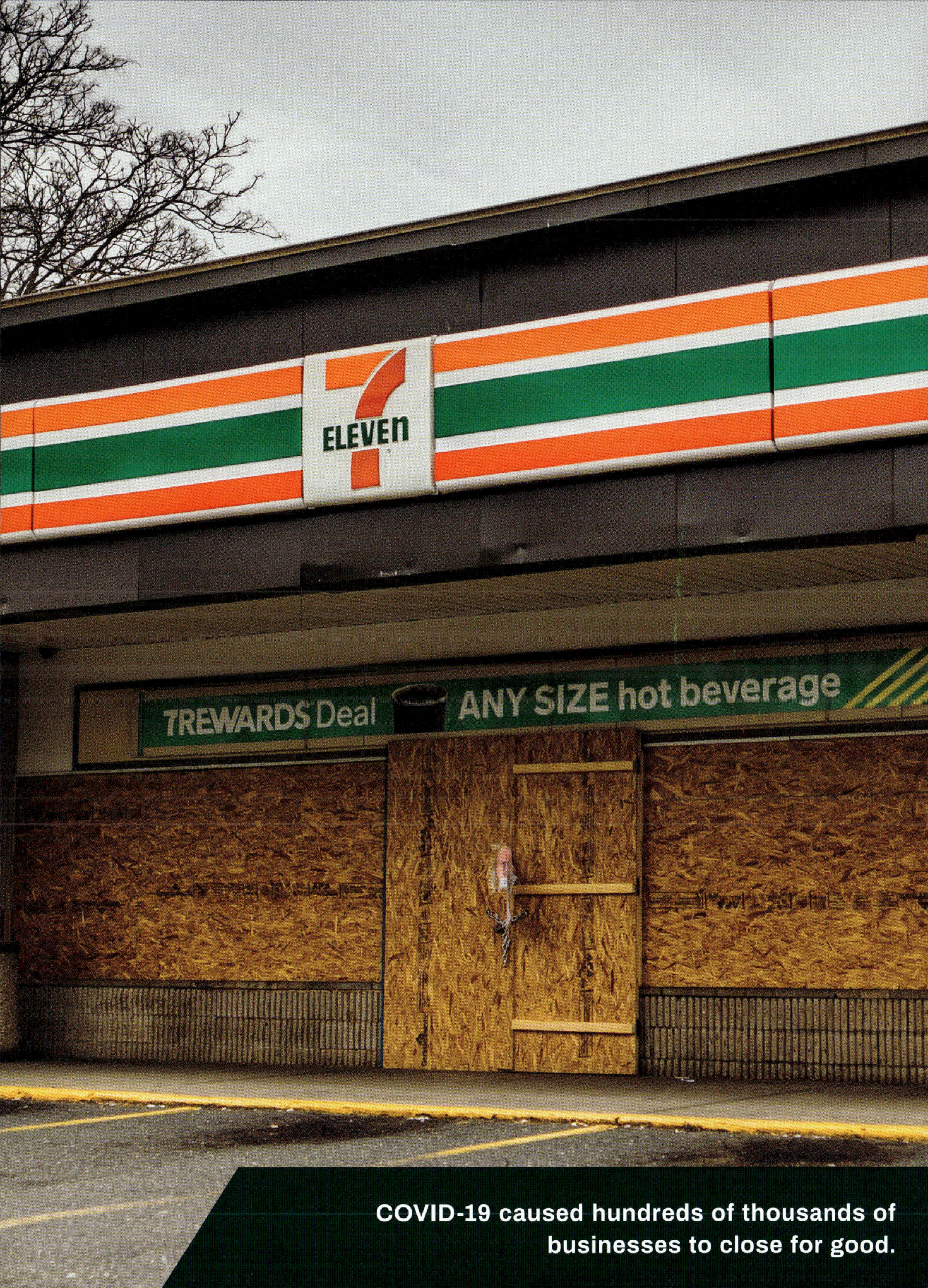

COVID-19 caused hundreds of thousands of businesses to close for good.

Loss of life was severe as well. By May 2023, there had been more than 765 million cases. Most people got better. But almost 7 million died.

During the pandemic, essential workers were more likely to struggle with mental health.

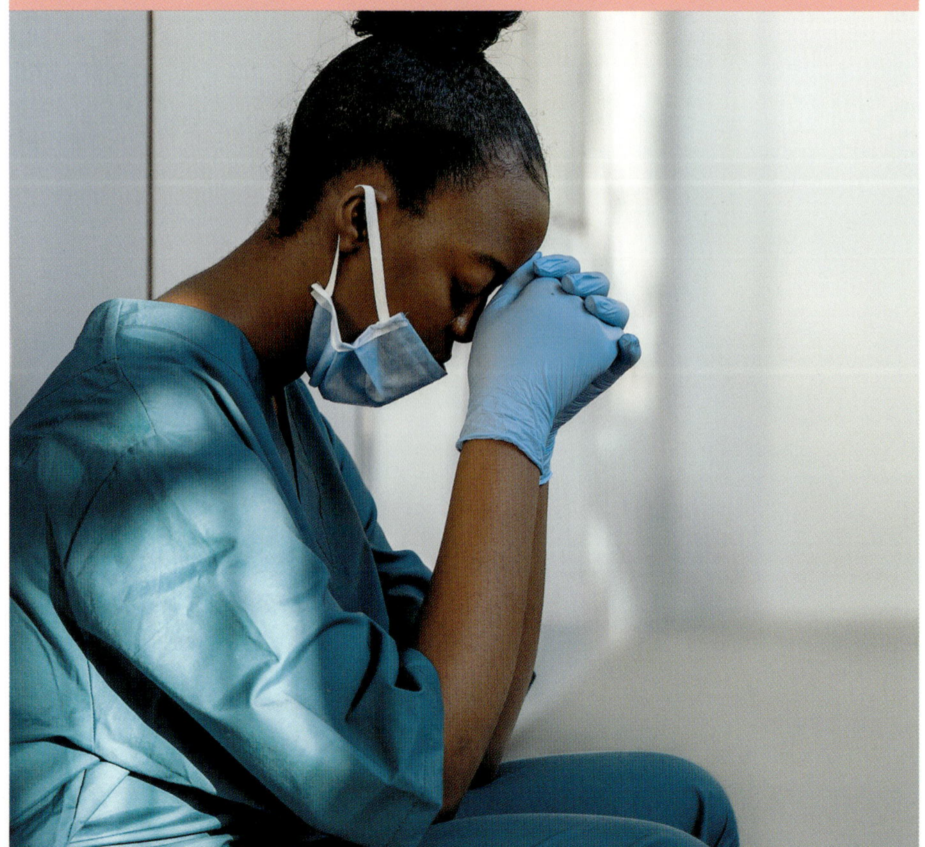

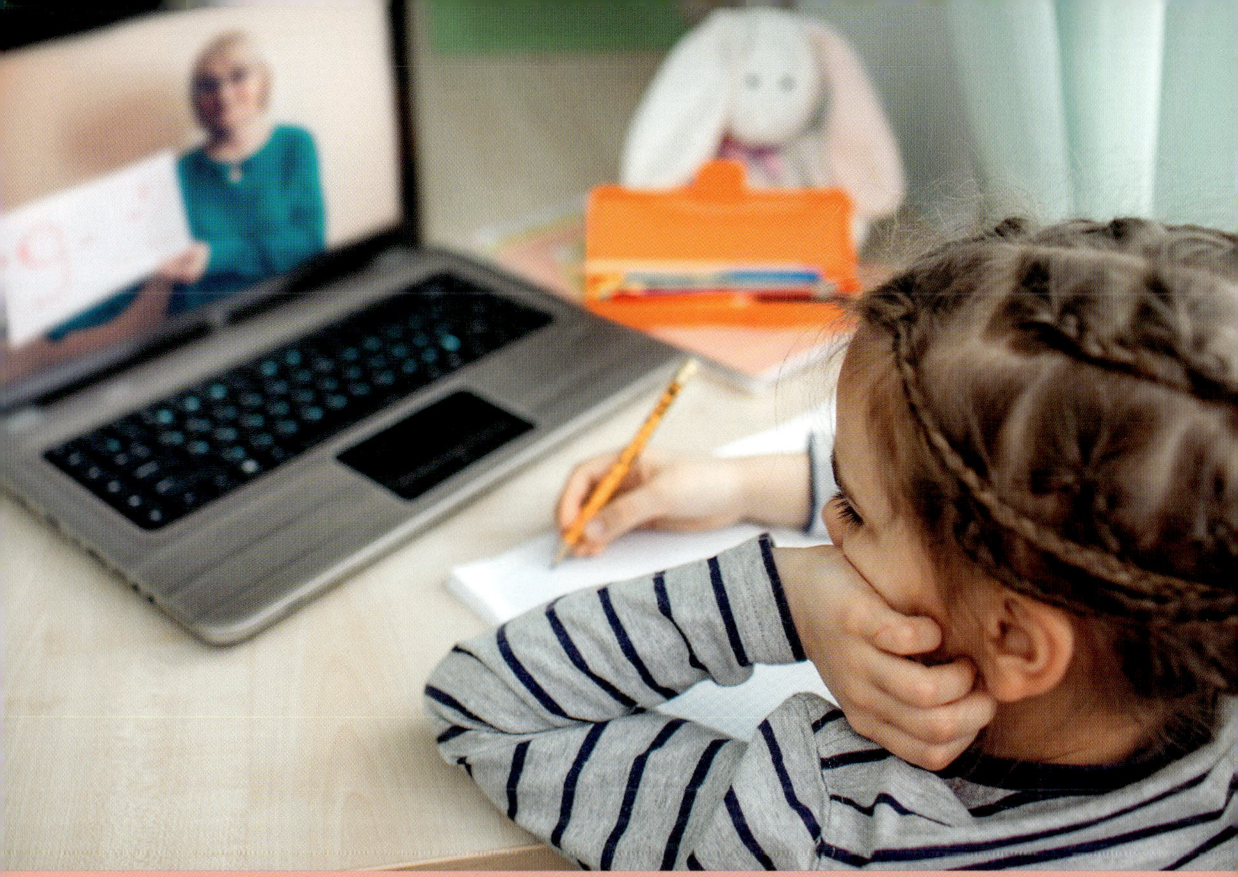

Some students struggled with online learning. Many fell behind in school.

MENTAL HEALTH

The pandemic affected mental health, too. Staying inside and away from others was difficult. People felt fear, stress, and grief. Many had friends or family members die.

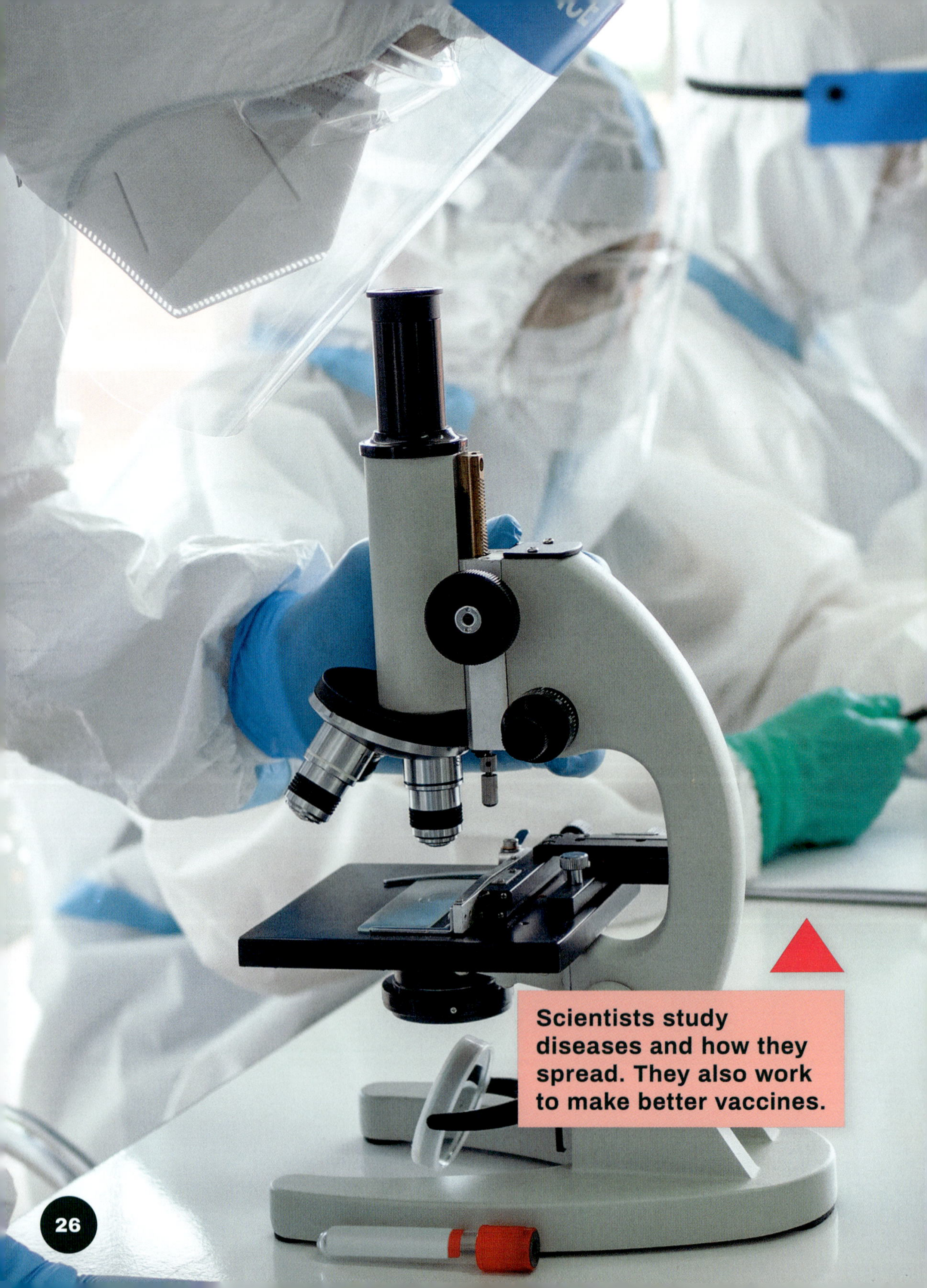

Scientists study diseases and how they spread. They also work to make better vaccines.

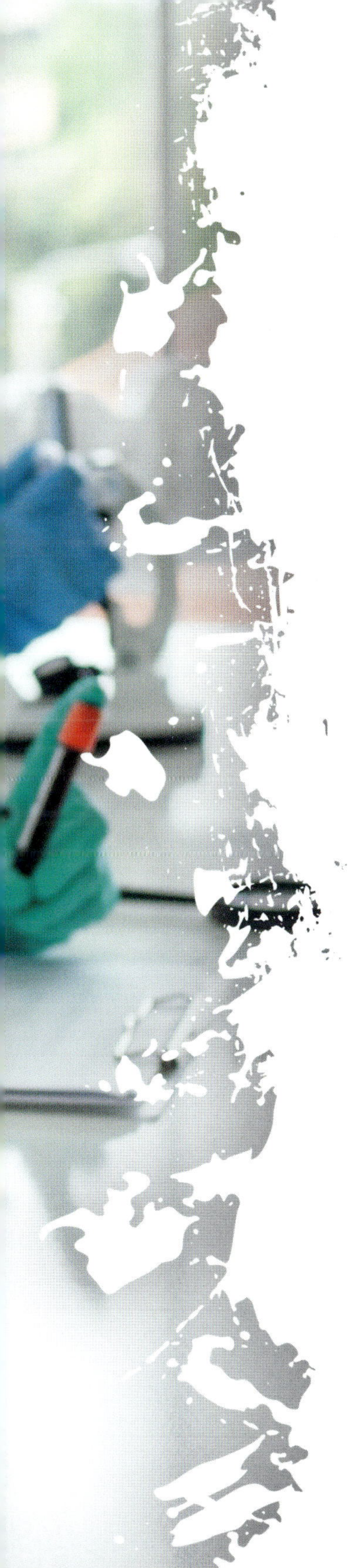

In May 2023, the pandemic was no longer an emergency. But governments and scientists kept working. They studied what happened. And they planned ways to protect people in the future.

FAST FACT
Some people's symptoms lasted for years. That was known as long COVID.

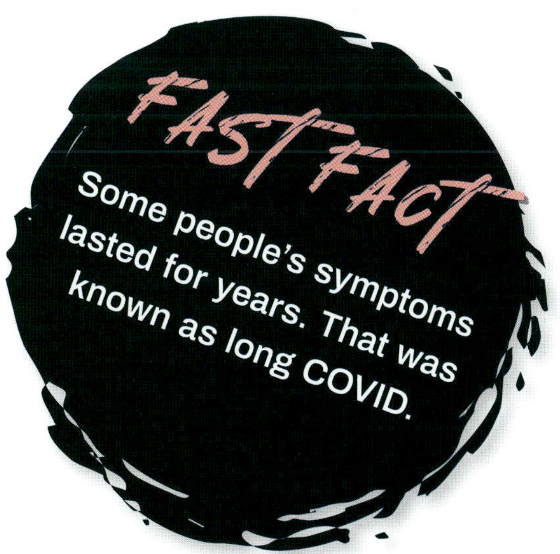

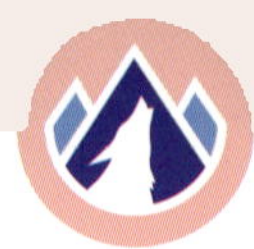

COMPREHENSION QUESTIONS

Write your answers on a separate piece of paper.

1. Write a few sentences describing the main ideas of Chapter 3.

2. Which method of slowing the pandemic's spread do you think was the most useful? Why?

3. When were the first COVID-19 vaccines ready?

- **A.** March 2020
- **B.** December 2020
- **C.** May 2023

4. How can quarantining help slow the spread of a disease?

- **A.** People who quarantine stop being sick.
- **B.** More people are exposed, so fewer get sick.
- **C.** Fewer people are exposed, so fewer get sick.

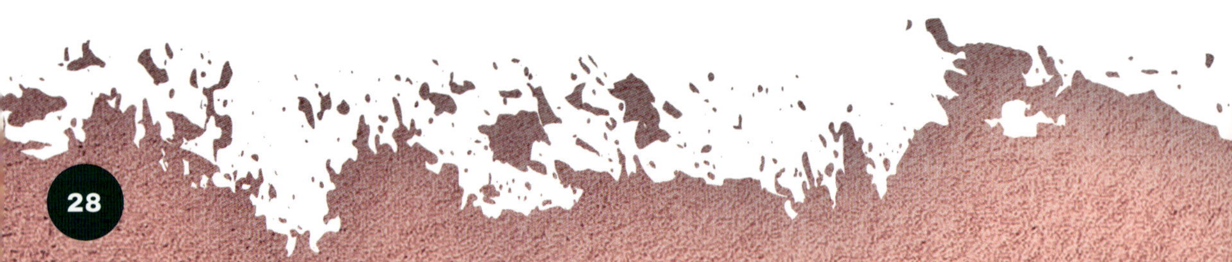

5. What does **positive** mean in this book?

*The test is **positive**. That means the girl has COVID-19.*

- **A.** giving good news
- **B.** finding signs of illness
- **C.** failing to work

6. What does **data** mean in this book?

*Testing and tracking helped scientists study COVID-19. They used the **data** to learn more about the virus.*

- **A.** places that people go for fun
- **B.** facts gathered to study something
- **C.** times of day or night

Answer key on page 32.

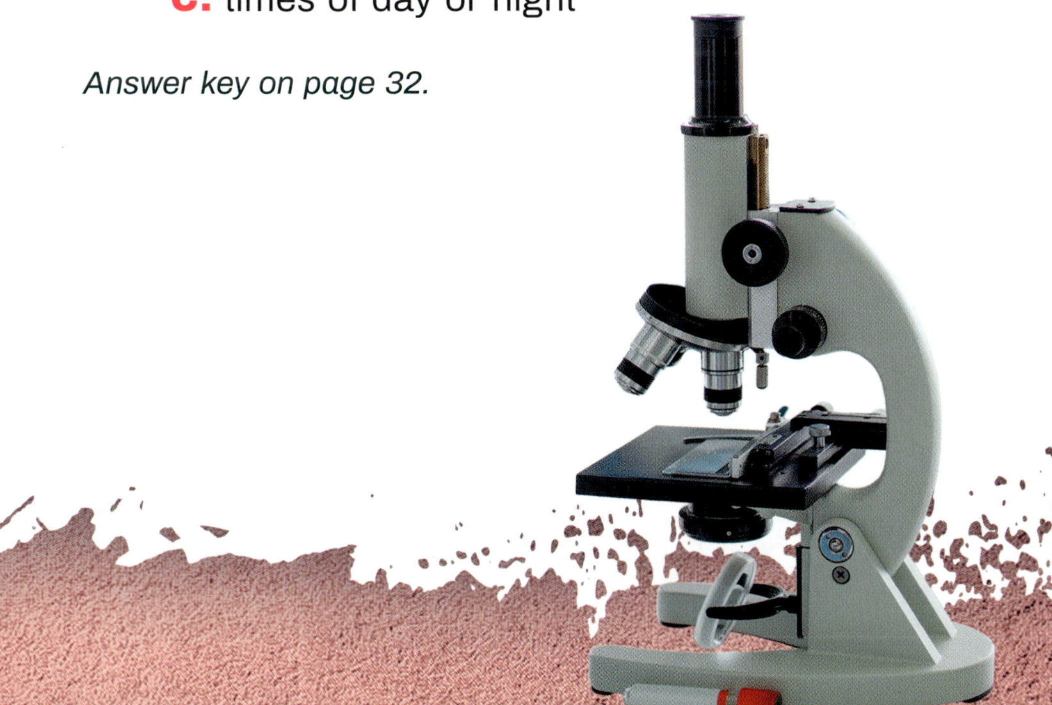

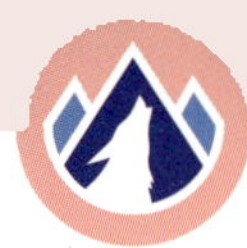

GLOSSARY

essential

Important or necessary.

exposed

Near someone with a disease that can be spread to others.

infectious diseases

Illnesses caused by germs getting into the body.

lockdowns

Times when people must stay in certain areas, such as inside their homes.

pandemic

A time when a disease spreads quickly around the world.

symptoms

Signs of an illness or disease.

vaccines

Substances that help a person's body fight a disease.

virus

A tiny substance that can cause illness in people and animals.

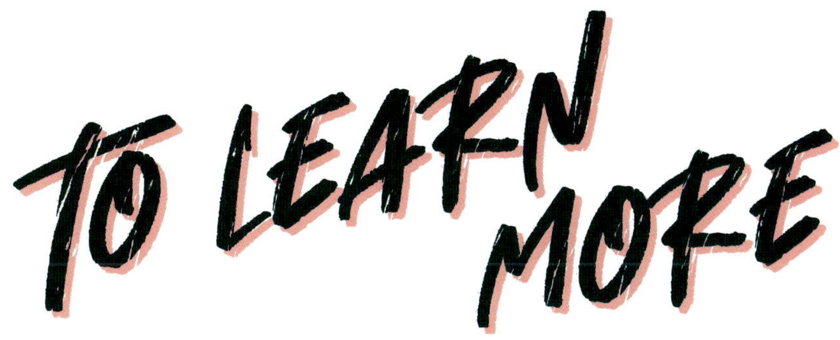

BOOKS

Abdo, Kenny. *COVID-19 Pandemic*. Minneapolis: Abdo Publishing, 2021.

Goldstein, Margaret J. *Understanding COVID-19*. Minneapolis: Lerner Publications, 2022.

Sommer, Nathan. *The Coronavirus Pandemic*. Minneapolis: Bellwether Media, 2022.

ONLINE RESOURCES

Visit **www.apexeditions.com** to find links and resources related to this title.

ABOUT THE AUTHOR

Trudy Becker lives in Minneapolis, Minnesota. She likes exploring new places and loves anything involving books.

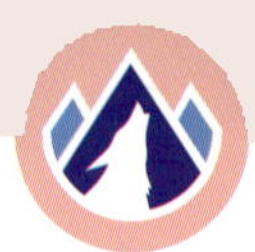

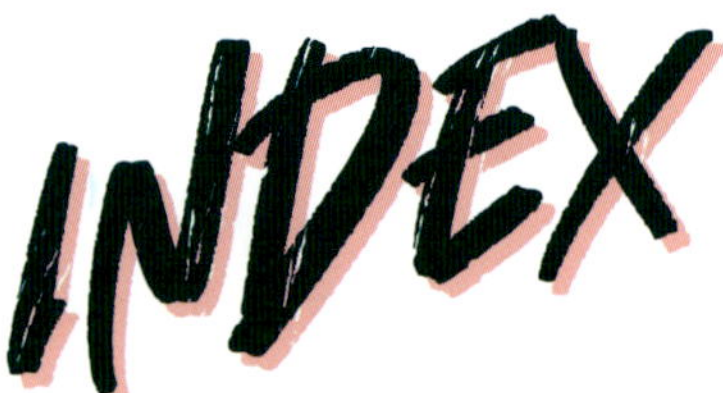

INDEX

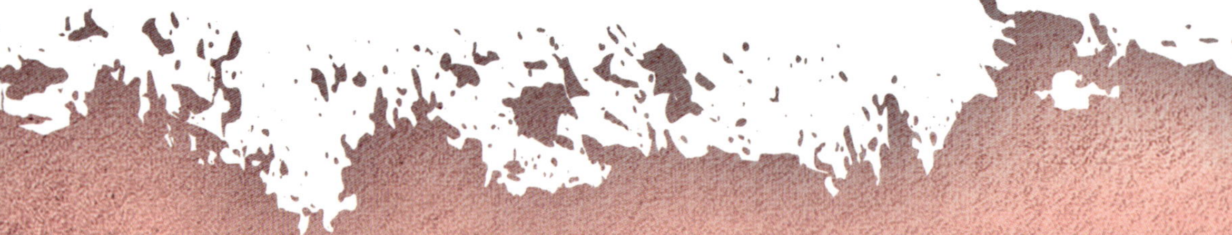

ANSWER KEY:
1. Answers will vary; 2. Answers will vary; 3. B; 4. C; 5. B; 6. B